NATTOKINASE FOR BEGINNERS

Unlocking Nattokinase A Comprehensive Guide To Heart Wellness Unveiling The Power Of Cardiovascular Health And Blood Circulation

Georgette Lockett

DISCLAIMER

The author of this book is not affiliated, associated, endorsed, sponsored, or approved by any company or individual. The views and opinions expressed in this book are solely those of the author and do not necessarily reflect the official policy or position of any entity.

The author hereby disclaims any relationship, collaboration, or partnership with any company or individual mentioned in this book. Any references to products, services, or individuals are provided for informational purposes only and should not be construed as an endorsement or recommendation.

Readers are advised to exercise their own judgment and discretion when applying the information provided in this book. The author shall not be held responsible for any actions taken by readers based on the content of this book.

This book is intended for general informational purposes only, and the author makes no representations or warranties of any kind, express or implied, about the completeness, accuracy, reliability, suitability, or availability of the information contained herein. Any reliance on the information in this book is at the reader's own risk.

The author reserves the right to update, change, or modify any information in this book without notice. It is the responsibility of the reader to verify any information before taking any actions based on the content of this book.

By reading this book, the reader acknowledges and agrees to the terms of this disclaimer.

Table of Contents

INTRODUCTION

Nattokinase is an enzyme that has a long history in Japanese culture and cuisine. Nattokinase, derived from natto, a traditional Japanese dish made from fermented soybeans, has gained worldwide attention for its potential health benefits.

Overview Of Nattokinase

At its core, nattokinase is an enzyme with fibrinolytic properties, which means it can degrade fibrin, a protein involved in blood clot formation. This enzyme was isolated from natto, a dish made by fermenting soybeans with Bacillus subtilis var. natto. The fermentation process turns the soybeans into a sticky, pungent, and stringy food that has been consumed for centuries in Japan.

Historical Background

Natto is thought to have been discovered accidentally centuries ago in ancient Japan. Soybeans are said to have been left to soak and ferment naturally during the warmer months, resulting in the creation of this distinct food. Natto became a staple in Japanese cuisine over time, valued not only for its flavor but also for its potential health benefits.

Importance And Benefits

Nattokinase is significant because of its ability to support cardiovascular health. According to research, its fibrinolytic properties may aid in the breakdown of blood clots, potentially lowering the risk of cardiovascular events such as heart attacks and strokes. Furthermore, its ability to promote healthy circulation by assisting the body's natural clot-dissolving processes is an important factor in its acceptance.

Nattokinase gained popularity outside of Japan during the twentieth century as scientific research focused on its enzymatic properties and potential health benefits. It has piqued the interest of researchers looking into natural alternatives for cardiovascular health and clot-related issues.

The introduction of nattokinase into the global market, whether as a supplement or as a functional food ingredient, has piqued the interest of health-conscious individuals looking for natural ways to improve heart health and overall well-being.

The historical significance of this enzyme, combined with its potential health benefits, has sparked increased interest and investigation into its mechanisms, efficacy, and broader applications beyond its traditional culinary use.

CHAPTER 1

Understanding Nattokinase

What Is Nattokinase?

Nattokinase is an enzyme generated from "natto," a fermented soybean dish popular in Japan. It has received a lot of attention for its potential health benefits, especially in cardiovascular health. Nattokinase has fibrinolytic activity, which means it can dissolve fibrin, a protein involved in blood clotting.

Source And Production

Nattokinase is primarily derived from natto, a popular Japanese food. Natto is produced by fermenting soybeans with the Bacillus subtilis bacterium. This bacterium produces nattokinase as a byproduct during the fermentation process.

After that, the enzyme is extracted from the natto and can be taken as a supplement.

Chemical Composition

Nattokinase's chemical structure includes a group of enzymes known as serine proteases. Serine proteases are essential for protein degradation. Nattokinase is classified as a serine protease because its active site contains a serine amino acid. The molecular weight of the enzyme is approximately 27 kDa.

Other components of nattokinase include peptides, which are short chains of amino acids. These peptides may aid in its biological activities and health-promoting properties.

Understanding the source, production, and chemical composition of nattokinase lays the groundwork for investigating its potential health benefits.

In the following chapters, we'll look at its various aspects, from its mechanisms of action to its applications in medicine and health.

CHAPTER 2

Mechanism Of Action

Nattokinase, an enzyme derived from natto, a traditional Japanese fermented soybean dish, has several remarkable properties that contribute to its health benefits, particularly in cardiovascular health.

Enzymatic Properties

1. Nattokinase is a serine protease, which is a type of enzyme that breaks down proteins. It specifically belongs to the subtilisin subfamily of serine proteases. This enzymatic property is critical in the enzyme's various biological activities within the human body.

2. Fibrinolytic Activity: One of nattokinase's most notable properties is its ability to degrade fibrin, a protein involved in blood clot formation. Nattokinase is a fibrinolytic enzyme that cleaves the peptide bonds in fibrin. This function is critical to the potential cardiovascular benefits.

Clot Dissolving Abilities

1. **Thrombolytic Effect:** According to research, nattokinase may have thrombolytic properties, which means it can dissolve blood clots. This ability is especially appealing to people who are prone to thrombotic conditions or are recovering from cardiovascular events such as heart attacks or strokes.

2. **Plasmin Activation:** Nattokinase aids in the activation of plasmin, an enzyme involved in fibrinolysis. It may help to prevent abnormal clot formation by enhancing the body's natural mechanisms for clot breakdown.

Impact On Cardiovascular Health

1. Nattokinase may help regulate blood pressure by promoting vasodilation (the widening of blood vessels) and supporting healthy blood flow, according to research. This effect is due to its ability to degrade fibrinogen, a precursor to fibrin that can affect blood viscosity.

2. **Cholesterol Modulation:** Some research suggests that nattokinase may play a role in cholesterol management. It has the potential to lower LDL cholesterol (the "bad" cholesterol) and support overall lipid profile balance, though more extensive research is needed to confirm this effect conclusively.

3. **Antioxidant and anti-inflammatory properties:** While nattokinase is best known for its fibrinolytic properties, it also has antioxidant and anti-inflammatory properties. These characteristics may contribute to its potential benefits in reducing

oxidative stress and inflammation, both of which are associated with cardiovascular disease.

The mechanisms of action of nattokinase point to its potential as a natural supplement for cardiovascular health. However, more research is needed, including clinical trials and long-term studies, to confirm its efficacy, safety, and appropriate dosage for therapeutic use.

CHAPTER 3

Health Benefits Of Nattokinase

Nattokinase, an enzyme derived from the traditional Japanese dish natto, has gotten a lot of attention because of its potential health benefits:

Improved Circulation And Blood Flow

- **Fibrinolytic Activity:** Nattokinase is well-known for its fibrinolytic activity, which involves the breakdown of fibrin, a protein involved in blood clotting. This action may help to prevent excessive clot formation and improve blood circulation.

- **Thrombolytic Effects:** Research suggests that Nattokinase may help prevent blood clot formation by promoting fibrinogen breakdown, lowering the risk of conditions such as deep vein thrombosis (DVT) or stroke.

Blood Pressure Regulation

• **Hypertension Management:** Research suggests that Nattokinase may help regulate blood pressure. Its ability to promote fibrinolysis may contribute to blood vessel dilation and, as a result, aid in the management of hypertension.

• **ACE Inhibitory Activity:** Some research suggests that Nattokinase may have ACE inhibitory effects, potentially contributing to blood pressure control by modulating blood vessel constriction.

Anti-Inflammatory Effects

• **Inflammation Reduction:** Nattokinase has been studied for its anti-inflammatory properties. It may help reduce inflammation markers, which may be beneficial in a variety of inflammatory conditions.

• **Cardiovascular Health:** Nattokinase may contribute to overall cardiovascular health by promoting healthy blood flow and supporting clot dissolution, potentially lowering the risk of heart-related issues.

- **Improved Vascular Health:** Improving circulation through the breakdown of blood clots may help to maintain vascular health and prevent conditions associated with poor blood flow.

- **Potential Benefits Other Than Cardiovascular Health:** Some studies suggest that there may be benefits other than cardiovascular health, such as supporting bone health and alleviating symptoms of certain skin conditions.

While several studies suggest these potential benefits, more research is needed to confirm and further understand the mechanisms and optimal use of Nattokinase for these health benefits. Individuals with pre-existing health conditions or those taking medications should seek the advice of a healthcare professional before incorporating Nattokinase supplements into their regimen, due to the potential for interactions and varying responses based on individual health statuses.

CHAPTER 4

Nattokinase And Cardiovascular Health

Role In Preventing Heart Diseases

Nattokinase, an enzyme derived from the Japanese fermented soybean dish "natto," has received attention for its potential role in cardiovascular health. One of its main mechanisms is fibrinolytic activity, or the ability to degrade fibrin, a protein involved in blood clotting. This may aid in the prevention and management of heart disease. Blood clots in the arteries can cause heart attacks or strokes. The ability of nattokinase to dissolve clots may help to reduce the risk of these conditions.

Potential Effects On Stroke Prevention

Stroke, which is frequently caused by blood clotting that prevents blood flow to the brain, is a major concern around the world.

According to research, Nattokinase's fibrinolytic properties may reduce the risk of ischemic strokes, the most common type caused by blood clots. Nattokinase may improve blood flow and reduce the risk of stroke by breaking down these clots.

Supporting Evidence And Research

Several studies have been conducted to investigate the effects of Nattokinase on cardiovascular health. Clinical trials and animal studies have yielded encouraging results. Nattokinase, for example, has been shown in studies to improve blood flow, lower blood pressure, and reduce blood clot formation. However, while these findings are encouraging, more extensive and rigorous research is required to establish its efficacy and safety.

In conclusion, Nattokinase, derived from natto, has fibrinolytic properties that may benefit cardiovascular health. Its ability to dissolve clots suggests that it could help prevent heart disease and reduce the risk of stroke. Nonetheless, additional well-controlled studies are required to fully understand its mechanisms, dosage, and long-term effects. Nattokinase shows promise, but its use as a cardiovascular health supplement requires more research and testing to confirm its efficacy and safety for widespread use.

CHAPTER 5

Nattokinase And Blood Clotting

Influence On Blood Clots And Fibrinolysis

Nattokinase, which is derived from the traditional Japanese dish natto, has gotten a lot of attention for its potential role in promoting cardiovascular health, particularly in terms of blood clotting and fibrinolysis. Fibrinolysis is the body's natural process for breaking down blood clots, and nattokinase is thought to aid in this process.

1. Activity in Fibrinolysis:

• *Fibrin Degradation:* Nattokinase is known for its fibrinolytic properties, which means it can break down fibrin, a protein involved in the formation of blood clots. Its primary component, the enzyme nattokinase, is responsible for this ability.

- *Plasmin Activation:* Nattokinase stimulates the activation of plasmin, an enzyme involved in the dissolution of fibrin. Plasmin works by cleaving fibrin into smaller fragments, preventing blood clot formation and growth.

Comparison With Traditional Blood Thinners

- **Natural Alternative:** Nattokinase is a natural alternative to traditional blood thinners such as aspirin and warfarin. It is made from fermented soybeans and is frequently preferred by people looking for alternatives to synthetic medications.

- **Broader Impact:** Unlike conventional blood thinners, which typically target a single step in the clotting cascade, nattokinase's action on plasmin activation allows it to affect multiple stages of clot formation and breakdown.

- **Less Side Effects:** Some research suggests that nattokinase may have fewer side effects than synthetic blood thinners. Individual responses may differ, so consulting with a healthcare professional is essential.

Safety Considerations

- **Dose-Dependent Effects:** The ability of nattokinase to promote fibrinolysis is frequently dose-dependent. Individuals with specific health conditions may require higher doses, and the appropriate dosage should be determined under the supervision of a healthcare provider.

- **Drug Interactions:** People who take anticoagulant medications or have bleeding disorders should use caution when considering nattokinase supplementation. To avoid potential interactions, it is critical to consult with a healthcare professional.

- **Monitoring and Adjustments:** Individuals incorporating nattokinase into their routine should monitor their clotting parameters regularly, especially if they are also taking prescription blood thinners. Medication dosage adjustments may be required under medical supervision.

Finally, the potential effect of nattokinase on blood clotting and fibrinolysis suggests that it may have applications in cardiovascular health. Individuals contemplating its usage, however, should do so under the supervision of a healthcare expert, who should examine their general health, current drugs, and individual reactions to supplementation.

CHAPTER 6

Usage And Dosage

Recommended Dosage Guidelines

Because of its possible cardiovascular advantages, nattokinase is often used as a dietary supplement. However, choosing the appropriate dose depends on the individual's health status and demands. While there isn't a standardized dosage endorsed universally, general recommendations range from 100 mg to 2,000 mg per day. It's crucial to follow the instructions on the supplement label or consult a healthcare professional to determine the appropriate dosage, especially if one is on other medications or has underlying health issues.

Forms Of Administration

Nattokinase is usually available in capsule or tablet form. Some nutritional supplements also provide it in powder form, making it easy to incorporate with beverages or meals. The bioavailability and efficacy could change depending on the formulation, therefore selecting a renowned brand with high-quality manufacturing standards is advised.

Precautions And Interactions

- **Blood Thinning Effect:** Nattokinase shows features that may help avoid excessive blood clotting. Individuals using anticoagulants or antiplatelet treatments should be careful since combining these medications with Nattokinase can enhance their effects, leading to an increased risk of bleeding. Consulting a healthcare physician before commencing Nattokinase supplements is crucial for people on blood-thinning drugs.

- **Surgery and Dental treatments:** Due to its possible blood-thinning effects, it's suggested to cease taking Nattokinase at least two weeks before planned surgeries or dental treatments to avoid the risk of excessive bleeding.

- **Pregnancy and nursing:** There is insufficient data on the safety of Nattokinase during pregnancy and nursing. It's encouraged for pregnant or breastfeeding persons to avoid Nattokinase supplementation unless prescribed and monitored by a healthcare practitioner.

- **Sensitive Reactions:** While allergies to Nattokinase are uncommon, those sensitive to soy or other components of fermented soybeans, from which Nattokinase is made, should avoid its usage.

Monitoring And Interactions

Regular monitoring of clotting parameters, particularly for those using Nattokinase in combination with other blood-thinning drugs, is critical. This helps guarantee that the combination does not lead to extremely thin blood and consequent bleeding issues.

• Always contact a healthcare practitioner before taking any new supplement, particularly if there are pre-existing health concerns or if you're currently on medication.

• Purchase supplements from trustworthy providers to assure quality and safety.

• Keep note of any side effects or bad reactions and quickly report them to a healthcare provider.

Nattokinase, a powerful enzyme generated from fermented soybeans, has received interest for its possible cardiovascular benefits. However, its use should be treated carefully, notably concerning its combination with blood-thinning drugs and associated negative effects. Adherence to authorized doses and adequate consultation with healthcare specialists may assist in safe and successful supplementing.

CHAPTER 7

Nattokinase In Traditional Medicine

Historical Use In Traditional Practices

Nattokinase has a deep history based on traditional Japanese medicine. Its roots extend back to natto, a classic Japanese meal made from fermented soybeans. Natto has been a mainstay in Japanese cuisine for generations, and it is thought that its intake adds to many health advantages. Nattokinase, the enzyme generated from the fermentation process of natto, has been identified for its potential therapeutic qualities.

In traditional Japanese medicine, natto has been utilized not only as a nutritional staple but also as a cure for numerous health ailments. The fermentation process is regarded to boost the bioavailability of minerals and bioactive substances, including nattokinase. Historical records show that natto was ingested for its purported cardiovascular advantages and its capacity to improve general well-being.

Cultural Significance

Nattokinase bears a cultural value in Japan, where it has been welcomed not just for its flavor but also for its possible health-promoting effects. The longstanding usage of nattokinase illustrates the profound relationship between culture, nutrition, and well-being in Japanese society.

In Japanese mythology and traditional beliefs, foods like natto and nattokinase are commonly connected with longevity and energy. The cultural relevance of nattokinase is ingrained in the belief that what people eat may impact their health and lifespan. The veneration for traditional treatments like nattokinase illustrates the holistic attitude to well-being evident in Japanese society.

Additionally, the incorporation of nattokinase into traditional medicine represents the knowledge of centuries past, when natural sources were studied for their possible curative capabilities. The cultural relevance of nattokinase goes beyond its nutritional qualities, reflecting a relationship between heritage, health, and the awareness of the natural world.

Understanding the historical usage of nattokinase in traditional Japanese medicine gives useful insights into its cultural background and the persistent belief in the health benefits obtained from natural, fermented sources. As current research continues to investigate the possibilities of nattokinase, appreciating its traditional origins adds depth to its expanding role in supporting health and well-being.

CHAPTER 8

Potential Side Effects

Nattokinase, derived from the traditional Japanese meal Natto, has attracted interest for its possible health advantages, notably in cardiovascular health. While it is usually regarded as safe for many persons, it is necessary to research possible side effects, adverse reactions, contraindications, and risk factors related to its usage.

Adverse Reactions

1. Sensitive Reactions: Although uncommon, some persons may be sensitive to soy, a main component in Natto, and subsequently, to nattokinase. Allergies may show as skin rashes, itching, swelling, or trouble breathing. Individuals with soy sensitivities should exercise caution and contact a healthcare practitioner before taking nattokinase supplements.

2. Digestive Issues: Some users may suffer moderate digestive discomfort, such as bloating, gas, or diarrhea. This may vary from person to person and could be impacted by the individual's digestive sensitivity.

Contraindications

1. Blood problems: Individuals with blood problems or those using anticoagulant drugs should check with their healthcare professional before using nattokinase. Nattokinase has inherent anticoagulant qualities, and its usage may increase bleeding difficulties.

2. Surgery and Dental treatments: Due to its anticoagulant effects, patients planning for surgery or dental treatments should notify their healthcare practitioners about their nattokinase usage. The supplement can raise the risk of bleeding during and after these operations.

Risk Factors

1. Pregnancy and nursing: Limited data available on the safety of nattokinase during pregnancy and nursing. As a precaution, pregnant and nursing persons should check with their healthcare practitioners before integrating nattokinase into their regimen.

2. Interaction with medicines: Nattokinase may interact with some medicines, such as anticoagulants (warfarin, heparin), antiplatelet drugs (aspirin, clopidogrel), and nonsteroidal anti-inflammatory drugs (NSAIDs). Combining nattokinase with these drugs may raise the risk of bleeding. It is vital for persons using these drugs to get advice from their healthcare providers before utilizing nattokinase supplements.

It is crucial for persons contemplating nattokinase supplementation to be aware of these possible adverse effects, contraindications, and risk factors.

Consulting with a healthcare practitioner before introducing nattokinase into one's routine is suggested, particularly for individuals with pre-existing health issues or those using drugs that may interact with nattokinase. Personalized medical guidance assures safe and successful usage based on individual health state and requirements.

CHAPTER 9

Research And Scientific Studies

Clinical Trials And Findings

Nattokinase, generated from fermented soybeans, has received interest owing to its possible health advantages, notably regarding cardiovascular health and blood coagulation. Numerous clinical studies have studied its effects:

1. **Cardiovascular Health:** Studies have studied Nattokinase's influence on several cardiovascular indicators. Research shows it may maintain healthy blood pressure levels by assisting in the breakdown of fibrin, a protein implicated in blood clot formation. Several investigations have shown its ability to enhance indicators related to cardiovascular well-being.

2. **Blood Clot Dissolution:** Clinical experiments have shown encouraging results in its capacity to break

and dissolve blood clots. Nattokinase's fibrinolytic characteristics, comparable to those of standard blood thinners, have been studied in several researches. Its mode of action includes the activation of plasmin, an enzyme responsible for clot breakdown.

3. Reduced Risk of Stroke and Heart Disease: Some research shows that frequent ingestion of Nattokinase can lower the risk of stroke and heart disease. This impact might be attributable to its capacity to maintain good blood flow and prevent clot formation.

Future Directions In Nattokinase Research

1. Clinical Validation: Further large-scale clinical studies are required to consolidate the reported benefits and define appropriate doses for particular health issues. More comprehensive investigations are necessary to validate past results and establish

Nattokinase’s effectiveness and safety characteristics.

2. Exploring Novel uses: Beyond cardiovascular health, researchers are studying possible uses in other areas, such as inflammation control, better circulation, and improving overall vascular health. Understanding its processes in these settings may create new options for therapeutic usage.

3. Bioavailability and Formulations: Research concentrating on increasing Nattokinase's bioavailability and stability will be helpful for its successful application in therapeutic interventions. Novel formulations and delivery techniques could increase its absorption and efficacy.

Peer-Reviewed Publications

A rising corpus of work in peer-reviewed publications has added to the knowledge of Nattokinase's potential advantages. These articles span a spectrum of investigations, from in vitro and animal models to human clinical trials. They present varied viewpoints on its methods of action, safety profiles, and prospective therapeutic uses.

CHAPTER 10

Incorporating Nattokinase Into Daily Life

Nattokinase, acclaimed for its possible cardiovascular benefits, has gained appeal as a dietary supplement. Understanding its assimilation into everyday life needs evaluating many facets: supplement types, lifestyle choices, and expert assistance.

Supplements And Products

Nattokinase supplements are available in numerous formats, including capsules, pills, powders, and in combination with other enzymes or cardiovascular support components. The decision frequently relies on personal preferences, dose needs, and the existence of any unique health issues. It's vital to purchase high-quality supplements from renowned producers to guarantee purity and effectiveness.

When adding Nattokinase into your regimen, evaluate the supplement's dose. The suggested dose may vary depending on individual health circumstances and the desired effect. Consulting a healthcare expert or a skilled nutritionist may give tailored advice on the correct form and dose.

Lifestyle Considerations

While Nattokinase supplements may be useful, they operate best as part of a holistic approach to health. A balanced diet, regular exercise, stress management, and proper sleep play essential roles in cardiovascular fitness. Incorporating heart-healthy meals like fruits, vegetables, whole grains, and lean meats with Nattokinase might boost its advantages.

Moreover, it's necessary to keep an active lifestyle. Regular physical exercise not only helps cardiovascular health but also complements the benefits of Nattokinase by boosting circulation and general well-being.

Stress management approaches such as meditation, yoga, or other relaxation activities may synergize with Nattokinase's potential advantages. Reducing stress levels is important for heart health and general well-being.

Consultation And Professional Guidance

Before beginning any supplement regimen, including Nattokinase, contacting a healthcare physician or a skilled practitioner is crucial. They may analyze individual health conditions, medicines, allergies, and any interactions. Especially for persons with existing medical problems or those using drugs, expert advice assures the safe and successful absorption of Nattokinase into their routine.

Regular health check-ups are vital while utilizing Nattokinase or any supplement long-term. Monitoring health metrics helps analyze the supplement's effectiveness and any possible changes in health status.

Integrating Nattokinase into everyday life demands attentive awareness of its supplements, lifestyle choices, and seeking expert help. By combining Nattokinase supplements with a heart-healthy lifestyle and individualized counsel, people might optimize its advantages for cardiovascular health. Always emphasize educated choices and contact healthcare specialists to ensure safe and effective use.

Conclusion

Recap Of Nattokinase Benefits

Throughout this investigation, we've explored the varied properties of Nattokinase, a powerful enzyme generated from fermented soybeans. Its therapeutic potential is fascinating, particularly in the domain of cardiovascular health. Key advantages noted include:

1. **Cardiovascular Health Enhancement:** Nattokinase's capacity to improve cardiovascular health by improving healthy circulation and perhaps lowering blood clot formation is notable.

2. **Blood Thinning Properties:** Unlike traditional blood thinners, Nattokinase exhibits the ability to alter clotting pathways without some of the undesirable effects associated with pharmacological treatments.

3. **Enzymatic Activity:** Its particular enzymatic characteristics contribute to its effectiveness in

breaking down fibrin and boosting the body's natural clot-dissolving activities.

Summary Of Key Findings

- **Mechanism of activity:** Nattokinase's enzymatic activity particularly targeting fibrin, the protein implicated in blood clot formation, sets it apart as a natural clot-dissolving agent.

- **Traditional and Modern Use:** From ancient origins in Japanese cuisine to its current use in supplements, Nattokinase has emerged as a potential help in supporting heart health.

- **Dose and Safety:** Understanding the optimal dose, modalities of administration, and possible interactions and precautions is vital for safe usage.

Nattokinase's development as a possible supplement for cardiovascular health is both hopeful and difficult. While evidence emphasizes its advantages, the subtleties around dose, safety, and its interaction with individuals’ distinct health profiles deserve additional inquiry. Its natural origins, along with its capacity to modify blood clotting pathways, provide an interesting route for comprehensive cardiovascular treatment.

As science continues to uncover the mysteries of Nattokinase, it is critical to approach its use with a balanced attitude, recognizing both its promise and the need for more study. The research of nature's medicinal abundance continues in the world of natural health supplements, and Nattokinase stands as a witness to that.

THE END

Printed in France by Amazon
Brétigny-sur-Orge, FR